Keto Meal Prep

How to Save $100 and 4 Hours A Week by Batch Cooking

I0146263

By Jason Michaels

Medical Disclaimer
This book is not intended as a substitute for the medical advice of physicians. The reader should regularly consult a physician in matters relating to his/her health and particularly with respect to any symptoms that may require diagnosis or medical attention.

Please consult your physician before starting any diet or exercise program.

Any recommendations given in this book are not a substitute for medical advice.

Table of Contents

- Mango Coconut Chicken Bowls
- Chicken Tikka Masala Prep Bowls
- Spinach, Tomato, and Bacon Muffin Tin Quiche
- Taco Scramble
- Chicken Sausage and Peppers
- Southwestern Chicken Burrito Bowls
- Skinny Joes With Tangy Slaw

- Mason Jar Recipes

  - Asian Chicken Mason Jar Salad
  - Yogurt and Granola Parfait
  - Zucchini Lasagna
  - Berry and Nuts Salad
  - Asian Noodle Salad
  - Mediterranean Salad
  - Feta and Shrimp Cobb Salad
  - BLT Salad
  - Rainbow Salad
  - Spinach, Tomato, Mozzarella Salad

- Dinner Recipes

  - Chipotle Turkey and Sweet Potato Chili
  - Avocado Bacon Garlic Burger
  - Chutney Cilantro Meatballs
  - Instant Pot Lamb Shanks
  - Cranberry Spice Pot Roast

- Garlic Pork and Kale
- Lemon Pepper Salmon
- Beef and Broccoli
- Shrimp With Zucchini Noodles
- Shrimp Taco
- Lemon Roasted Salmon With Sweet Potatoes and Broccolini

- Dessert Recipes

  - Cinnamon Apples
  - Stuffed Peaches
  - Blackberry Curd
  - Cinnamon Pecan Chia Bars
  - Chocolate Coconut Bites
  - Oatmeal Energy Bars

- Fat Bomb Recipes

  - Walnut Orange Chocolate Bombs
  - Mini Lemon Tart Bombs
  - Cinnamon Roll Bomb Bars
  - Macadamia Chocolate Fudge Bombs
  - Peanut Butter Chocolate Bombs
  - Savory Mediterranean Fat Bombs
  - Bacon Guac Bombs
  - Salmon Bombs
  - Jalapeno and Cheese Bombs
  - Pizza Bombs

Introduction

Welcome and thank you for purchasing a copy of
Keto Meal Prep.

The world we live in today is all about hustling to
the next opportunity and bustling through the
inevitable daily to-do list. While we are succeeding
in our careers and family life, we are failing our
health by fueling our bodies with fatty convenience
store snacks, and fast food eats loaded with extra
sugars and carbs.

Now is not the time to blame yourself but realize
that you only have one body in this lifetime and you
need to begin treating it like the beautiful temple of
life it is! But how does someone who is constantly
busy and on-the-go eat healthier? Well, I am glad
you asked!

The chapters within this book hold two incredible
sources of getting your health back on track into
one jam-packed book of valuable information and
recipes! Let me introduce you to the ketogenic diet,
paired with the awesome convenience and power of
meal prepping!

The following chapters will discuss what the ketogenic diet is and how it can help you get your life back on track and feeling your best! But the best part of this book will teach you the basics of meal prepping and how it can drastically change the way you fuel your body; with meal prep, there are no excuses when it comes to choosing healthier meal choices because you already did all the work yourself!

Thanks again for your interest in how meal prepping on the ketogenic diet can change your life! Every effort was made to ensure it is full of as much useful information as possible, please enjoy!

Chapter 1: Brief Overview of the Keto Diet

This is a high-fat diet that this is low in carbs and moderate in protein consumption. The ketogenic is based on the metabolic state that you aim to get your body into, known as *ketosis.*

When your body is successfully in a ketosis state, the liver produces ketones, which become your body's main source of energy. The core of the keto is based around the idea that the human body was created to run better as a fat burner rather than a burner of sugar and carbs for energy. The ketogenic diet reverses the way in which your body functions in a positive manner. This means that it has the power to totally change your perspective on healthy nutrition!

Fat Torch Versus Sugar Burner

When you consume items that are high in carbs, such as that daily morning donut, your body has to create insulin and glucose to break it down:

- *Insulin* is created to help process the glucose in the bloodstream by transporting it throughout the body.

- *Glucose* is a molecule that is easily converted by the body as an energy source.

When glucose is the body's primary source of energy, fats are not needed, which means they are stored, also known as that pesky excess weight you want to rid yourself of. When your body uses all its glucose, your brain signals you to reach for a snack, which is typically unhealthy such as chips or candy.

This is where the ketogenic diet has the power to reverse the effects of unhealthy eating by transforming your body into a fat burner instead of a sugar burner. When you lower your consumption of carbohydrates, your body then tries to find another energy source, which is when your body enters ketosis.

When your body reaches the state of ketosis, fat cells release any water that they had been storing and the fat cells can make an entrance into the bloodstream and go to the liver. This is essentially the goal of the keto diet. Despite popular belief, you cannot enter ketosis by starving your body, but rather by not consuming carbohydrates.

Keto Diet Benefits

- More effective weight loss
- Improved cholesterol levels
- Decrease in insulin levels
- Improved blood sugar levels
- Elimination of diabetes precursors
- Decrease in the development of diseases like Parkinson's and Alzheimer's
- Treatment for cancer and growth of tumors
- Treatment for reducing symptoms of epilepsy
- Healthier skin

Foods to Avoid

- *Sugary foods*: cake, soda, candy, fruit juice, ice cream, etc.

- *Grains and starches*: anything wheat and corn-based produce such as pasta, rice, and cereals

- *Fruit*: most fruits excluding berries

- *Beans and legumes*: peas, lentils, chickpeas, kidney beans, etc.

- *Root vegetables and tubers*: carrots, parsnips, potatoes, etc.

- *Condiments*

- *Unhealthy fats*: vegetable oils, mayonnaise, etc.

- *Alcohol*

- *Anything labeled "sugar-free," "diet," or "low-carb"*: these items contain sugar alcohols that can greatly affect the success of reaching ketosis

Food to Embrace

- *Meat*: red meat, chicken, steak, turkey, sausage, ham, bacon, etc.

- *Fish*: salmon, trout, tuna, and mackerel

- *Cream and butter*: Grass-fed is the best

- *Nuts and seeds*: chia seeds, almonds, pumpkin seeds, walnuts, flaxseeds, etc.

- *Healthy oils*: extra virgin olive, coconut, avocado, etc.

- *Herbs and spices*

- *Low-carb vegetables*: green veggies, tomatoes, avocados, onions, peppers, etc.

Chapter 2: Why You Should Be Meal Prepping

There are many people that aspire to live a healthier lifestyle but have no idea where to start or have no time to spare. Eating healthy is one thing, but following through with your health and fitness goals and staying consistent is challenging.

When you have your hands full navigating life, cooking all our own meals can feel impossible, and the temptations of hitting up a fast food joint seem like an easier option.

If you are ready to reach your fitness goals, stop spending extraordinary amounts of money on junk food, then your new best friend is meal prepping!

What is Meal Prepping?

Meal prepping is planning, preparing, and packaging snacks and meals for the upcoming week with the idea of portion control and clean eating in mind. No right or wrong way happens to meal prep, which makes it a great dieting alternative for busy bees to personalize to fit into their daily schedule.

The goal of meal prepping is to save substantial time slaving away in the kitchen while having access to healthier meal options throughout the week. You simply dedicate time to planning your meals and cooking their components. Besides that, you will become *amazed* at the difference meal prepping will make in your day to day life!

Reasons Why You Should Be Meal Prepping

Effective weight loss

When you plan your meals in advance, you will know what you are putting into your body. A meal prep routine lets you control how many calories you consume, which is essential for weight loss.

Saves money

Despite popular belief, eating healthy doesn't have to be pricey. Purchasing things in bulk and taking advantage of your freezer is the key. You know exactly what to buy instead of purchasing ingredients you don't need. Plus, with meals already made, you will save a _ton_ of money on fast food meals - up to $100 a week in some cases.

Shopping is simpler

Once you plan your week's meals, grocery shopping will be a breeze since you will have a list to stick to instead of wandering around the store.

Learn portion control

Meal prep teaches you how to balance what you put inside your body. When you pack your meals in containers, it keeps you from reaching for more food that you don't need. This is essential if you want to lose weight; meal prepping allows you to control the nutrients and calories you eat.

Less waste

Meal prepping lets you utilize all your ingredients for the week before they go bad! This is a much better alternative than trashing expensive produce before you have a chance to eat it.

Saves time

While you will need to set time aside to prepare your meals, you will end up saving time in the long run. Think about it; how much time do you spend with the fridge open? How much time do you waste making a decision of what to eat just to become a victim of tempting convenience foods? With meal prep, meals are prepared ahead of time, requiring you to remove from the fridge and nuke them in the microwave. Easy!

Investment in your health

When you can pick what you are going to stuff your face with ahead of time, you have ample time to make much healthier decisions. The benefits of eating cleaner are endless! Good nutrition is everything, especially if you are looking to fit into that bikini for the summer!

Strengthens willpower

Once you become accustomed to eating healthier, you will find that you no longer crave sugar and carbs. When you have a consistent routine of eating better, you will turn down unhealthy food choices much easier.

Reduces stress

Stress directly impacts your immune system, which can cause you to experience digestive issues, lack of quality sleep, and many more negative side effects. Coming home from work and having a meal ready to eat takes away that everyday stress!

Adds variety to your diet

Once you get the hang of meal prepping, you will feel more confident to try new recipes with new ingredients. Your taste buds will receive a variety of flavor daily.

Chapter 3: How to Avoid the 10 Most Common Meal Prep Mistakes

The way you approach meal prepping will make a world of difference when it comes to successfully implementing it into your everyday life. There are many tips out there regarding choosing recipes, shopping, and bringing it all together to create a week's worth of delicious eats.

However, you need to be aware of the things that could potentially go wrong and be knowledgeable of solutions to avoid meal prep pitfalls.

Mistake 1: Not giving yourself enough time to plan

Meal planning takes time and cannot happen in an hour. When you plan, shop, and prep as soon as you can, you are not giving yourself a sufficient amount of time to process everything, which can make it more of a stressful experience than it has to be.

- *Solution:* Allow yourself ample time to plan meals, especially as a beginner. Set aside 2 to 3 hours per week. Take advantage of the weekend to spread out planning, shopping, and prepping of meals. This will allow prepping to feel like a sustainable task that you can do for months to come. An easy way to do this at first is to make a meal calender for the upcoming week. This will help you plan efficiently and avoid wasting food.

Mistake 2: Not choosing the best recipes for your personal needs

To ensure that meal prepping works the best for you and your lifestyle, you need to understand the importance of what your body needs from the recipes you choose. If you pick a bunch of recipes that don't come close to the criteria, you will be hungry and unsatisfied.

- **Solution:** Choose recipes based on the meals you *need.* While this seems obvious, many people overlook this. Create a list of what you want recipes to do for you.

    o Need recipes to be 30 minutes or less?
    o Are you a vegetarian?
    o What ingredients do you have that need to be used?

Mistake 3: Being unrealistic and too ambitious

Meal planning should be viewed as a marathon, not a sprint to the finish. You will feel super inspired at the start of your meal prep journey, but once you start to get into the depths of planning, you can become easily overwhelmed. You need to ensure that your prep schedule matches your regular schedule so that you can sustain it.

- **Solution:** Begin by creating defined goals and assessing your daily routine and schedule; this will help you to find what is realistic for *you.* Start small and start prepping two to three nights per week. This will give you the opportunity to figure out what works and what doesn't and allows you to tweak it to your liking.

Mistake 4: Not stocking the pantry

Experienced meal planners know how essential it is to always have meal basics on hand. If you fail to keep a good supply of staple items, you will miss all the benefits of meal planning and will likely become susceptible to temptation.

- *Solution:* Stock your pantry with all the basics that you can use time and time again in a variety of recipes:

    - Canned goods
    - White wine vinegar
    - Pepper, salt, and other spices
    - Canned tomatoes
    - Natural sweeteners (agave, maple, and honey)
    - Coconut milk
    - Olive oil
    - Stock
    - Etc.

Even on the days, you feel like you have nothing to consume, those basic components can help you create a yummy frittata, a delicious three-ingredient entre, or a one-pot wonder.

Mistake 5: Not searching for items that need to be used up

Before you head to the store, take an inventory of ingredients you already have in your kitchen and make use of leftover components you have. It's a simple step that helps you to prevent waste and saves you money.

- *Solution:* Before choosing recipes and making a grocery list, look in your cupboards, pantry, and fridge for food that needs to be used first. Turn those greens into a tasty side before going bad or thaw that pack of chicken to create a delicious main course.

Mistake 6: Not jotting down recipes

Meal prepping is all about being organized is you want to be successful. If you fail to save or write down recipes you have enjoyed, you will fall off track and become overwhelmed.

- *Solution:* Stay organized by keeping track of recipes that you have enjoyed and new ones you want to try out. It doesn't have to be fancy; could be a scrap piece of paper or on a whiteboard in your kitchen.

Mistake 7: Not taking inventory before shopping

Once you have picked your recipes for the week, you need to see what items you already have in your pantry. This is a closely tied mistake to not seeing the ingredients that need to be used before going bad.

- **Solution:** Before heading to the store, double check your recipe and the list of ingredients. Check your kitchen to ensure you don't have any of the components already so that you prevent overbuying.

Mistake 8: Skipping pre meal prep

Pre meal prepping is obviously an essential part of meal prep; this is small tasks like organizing ingredients and labelling containers. This gives your future self a giant hand. If you skip it, you are hurting yourself and leaves more work to do on the weekends.

- **Solution:** Set aside 30 minutes to an hour of prep each evening. This will make weekend meal prep a heck of a lot more efficient.

Mistake 9: Trying new recipes each day

I highly encourage you to try new recipes, but it's also important to go about eating a new variety of foods in a strategic way. When you fill up the whole week with brand new recipes, it can become very overwhelming and hard to sustain over a long period of time.

- *Solution:* Don't throw new recipes to the side but <u>build your meal plan</u> around recipes you know and then add 1 or 2 new recipes per week. This will help your taste buds from becoming bored and will also strengthen your recipe collection.

Mistake 10: Failing to have a backup plan

Even the most experienced meal preppers are bound to get stuck at work or have evenings where they are not feeling like consuming the dinner they planned out. Having a plan B is essential to stay the course.

- *Solution:* Have a good backup plan and have recipes in your back pocket that you know how to make. These will be very simple and can be made quickly, such as an omelet.

Chapter 4: Delicious Keto Recipes

The following sections withhold a wide array of delicious, easy-to-make keto meal prep recipes that you will certainly want to keep in that back pocket of yours! With these recipes, you will have fewer excuses when it comes to fueling your body in a way that makes you feel better both inside and out!

Breakfast Recipes

Greek Egg Bake

Protein: 15g Fat: 11g Net Carbs: 5g Calories: 175 Fiber: 9g

Ingredients:

- ¼ cup sun-dried tomatoes
- ½ cup feta cheese
- ½ tsp. oregano
- 1 cup chopped kale
- 12 eggs

Instructions:

1. Ensure your oven is preheated to 350 degrees.
2. With the foil, line a baking sheet and with the nonstick spray, spray well.
3. Whisk the eggs and then stir in the oregano, feta cheese, tomatoes, and kale.

4. In the sheet, pour the egg mixture. Then, bake the mixture for 25 minutes.

5. Let it cool and slice.

Can be served right away or kept in the fridge for 4 to 5 days.

Turmeric Scrambled Egg Meal Prep

Protein: 29g Fat: 18g Net Carbs: 6g Calories: 216 Fiber: 11g

Ingredients:

- ½ tsp. dried parsley
- 1 cup steamed broccoli
- 2 tbsps. coconut milk
- 2 tsp. dried turmeric
- 4 eggs
- 8 pre-cooked sausages

Instructions:

1. With the nonstick spray, grease a frying pan and then place it over medium heat setting.

2. Whisk the turmeric, parsley, milk, and eggs together with a pinch of the pepper and salt.

3. In the frying pan, slowly pour the mixture of eggs. Then cook well for 2 to 3 minutes, stirring the mixture constantly to break the eggs apart.

4. Flip the eggs and cook for another couple minutes till you reach the desired texture.

5. Add the eggs to two meal prep containers and add the veggies and sausage to the containers.

Can be refrigerated for up to 5 days.

Three-Ingredient Cauliflower Hash Browns

Protein: 7g Fat: 12g Net Carbs: 3.2g Calories: 164 Fiber: 2g

Ingredients:

- ¼ tsp. cayenne pepper
- 1 egg
- ¼ tsp. garlic powder
- ¾ cup shredded cheddar cheese
- ½ tsp. salt
- 1 head of cauliflower
- 1/8 tsp. pepper

Instructions:

1. Ensure your oven is preheated to 400 degrees. Grease a tray with the nonstick spray.

2. Grate the head of the cauliflower. For 3 minutes, place in the microwave and allow to cool. Ring out excess water with the cheesecloth or paper towels.

3. Place the cauliflower with the remaining ingredients and stir well to combine.

4. On a greased tray, form the mixture into square hash browns.

5. Bake for 15 to 20 minutes.

6. Let it cool for 10 minutes.

7. Serve it warm or place into the meal prep containers.

Can be refrigerated for 4 to 5 days.

Vegan Egg Muffins

Protein: 13g Fat: 9g Net Carbs: 4.1g Calories: 143 Fiber: 6g

Ingredients:

- ¼ cup coconut milk
- ½ thinly sliced sweet onion
- ½ tsp. dried oregano or 1 tsp. fresh oregano
- ¾ cup chopped red bell peppers
- ¾ tsp. sea salt
- 1 ½ cup fresh spinach
- 8-ounce pork breakfast sausage
- 1 tbsp. extra virgin olive oil
- 9 eggs

Instructions:

1. Ensure your oven is preheated to 350 degrees. Grease a muffin tin.
2. Sauté the ground sausage, breaking up as it cooks.
3. When halfway cooked, add a tablespoon of the olive oil, along with the oregano, pepper,

and onions. Sauté the mixture till the onions turn into translucent.

4. Cover the pan after adding the spinach. Cook for 30 seconds and then toss the mixture. Spinach should be wilted. Take the pan off the heat.
5. Mix the eggs in a bowl with the milk, pepper, and salt, whisking till well beaten.
6. To the eggs, add the cooked sausage and veggie mixture and mix till well combined.
7. In a muffin tin, put the mixture evenly.
8. Bake for 18 to 20 minutes.

Refrigerate for up to 4 days and frozen for up to 2 months.

Turkey Chorizo Breakfast Sandwich

*Protein: 29g Fat: 11g Net Carbs: 8g Calories: 203
Fiber: 5g*

Ingredients:

Turkey Chorizo:

- ¼ tsp. cayenne pepper
- 1 tsp. coriander
- ¼ tsp. dried thyme
- ¼ tsp. cinnamon
- ½ tsp. dried oregano
- ¼ tsp. pepper
- ¼ tsp. onion powder
- 1 tbsp. cumin
- 1 tsp. fennel seeds
- 1 tbsp. paprika
- 1 tsp. sea salt
- 1/8 tsp. cloves, ground
- 1-pound turkey breast, lean ground
- 1 tsp. garlic powder

Breakfast Sandwich:

- ¼ avocado
- 1 cooked turkey chorizo patty
- 1 egg
- 1 whole wheat English muffin

Instructions:

1. *TO make the chorizo:* In a bowl, add the turkey and spices. Mix them well with your clean hands. Create 16 even-sized portions and make them into ¼-inch patties.
2. Cook the chorizo patties in a greased skillet till the patties turn brown.
3. *To make a sandwich:* Spray a skillet and add the egg. Cook to your preference.
4. Toast your English muffin.
5. Serve the muffin topped with one chorizo patty, eggs, and avocado.

Freeze the remaining patties to enjoy throughout the week.

Banana Strawberry Baked Oatmeal

*Protein: 14g Fat: 16g Net Carbs: 7g Calories: 154
Fiber: 11g*

Ingredients:

- 2 eggs
- ¼ cup pure maple syrup
- ½ tsp. salt
- 1 ½ cup chopped strawberries + more to serve
- 1 tsp. cinnamon
- 2 tsp. vanilla extract
- 3 cups almond milk
- 3 mashed/ripe bananas
- 4 cups oats, old-fashioned
- 1 tsp. baking powder

Instructions:

1. Ensure your oven is preheated to 350 degrees. Grease a baking dish.
2. Whisk the salt, baking powder, cinnamon, vanilla, maple syrup, milk, eggs, and banana together well.

3. Mix in the oats. Gently fold in the strawberries.
4. In the prepared dish, pour the mixture. Then, bake the mixture for 35-40 minutes till the oatmeal sets.
5. Before serving, allow it to sit for 5 minutes. Then, serve the topping with more chopped strawberries.

Leftovers can be refrigerated for 3 days.
Simply reheat the oatmeal with a bit of the almond milk and top with desired fruit if you so choose.

Banana Muffins

Calories: 134 Protein: 11g Net Carbs: 9.8g Fiber: 9g Fat: 4g

Ingredients:

- ¼ tsp. salt
- 1 tsp. vanilla extract
- ½ tsp. baking soda
- ½ cup unsweetened applesauce
- 1 ½ cup ripe bananas
- 3 tbsps. olive oil
- 1 tsp. baking powder
- 1 egg
- 1 1/3 cup wheat flour, whole

Instructions:

1. Ensure your oven is preheated to 375 degrees. Grease a muffin tin well.
2. Light beat the egg and then add the bananas, mashing well. Stir the remaining components, minus the flour.
3. Then add the flour, stirring gently till well combined. DON'T OVERMIX.
4. In the muffin tin, pour the batter.

5. Then, bake the batter for 22 minutes.

Muffins can either be refrigerated for 7 days or frozen for 3 months.

Vanilla Cinnamon Protein Bites

Protein: 2g Fat: 9g Net Carbs: 4.2g Calories: 112 Fiber: 3g

Ingredients:

- ¼ - 1/3 cup nut butter of choice (the creamier, the better!)
- ¼ - 1/3 cup pure maple syrup
- ¼ cup vanilla protein powder
- ½ cup almond meal
- ½ - 1 tsp. vanilla extract
- ¾ cup quick oats
- 1 tbsp. cinnamon

Instructions:

1. Grind the oats in your food processor and pour them into a mixing bowl. Add the nut butter, cinnamon, protein powder, and almond meal to the bowl, stirring well.
2. Pour in the vanilla and syrup, combining well with your clean hands.
3. With the parchment paper, like a cookie sheet, roll the mixture making 1 ½-inch balls and place on the lined sheet.

4. Freeze for 20 to 30 minutes and then place in a Ziploc baggie.
5. Dust the balls with the vanilla protein and cinnamon.

Can be refrigerated for 3 weeks or frozen for up to 6 months.

Low-Carb Breakfast Pizza

Protein: 19g Fat: 16g Net Carbs: 7.2g Calories: 307 Fiber: 5g

Ingredients:

- ¼ tsp. pepper
- ½ cup heavy cream
- ½ tsp. salt
- 1 cup shredded cheese of choice
- 12 eggs
- 2 cups sliced peppers
- 8 ounces of sausage

Instructions:

1. Ensure your oven is preheated to 350 degrees.
2. Microwave the peppers for 3 minutes.
3. In a cast iron skillet, brown the sausage. Set to the side.
4. Mix the pepper, salt, cream, and eggs together and place in the skillet.
5. Cook for 5 minutes till the sides begin to become firm.

6. Place the skillet in the oven and back for 15 minutes. Then, remove the skillet from the oven.
7. To the skillet, add the cheese, peppers, and sausage and then for 3 minutes, place it under the broiler.
8. Allow to sit for 5 minutes to cool. Devour right away or split between the meal prep containers.

Can be refrigerated for 5 days or frozen for 60 days.

Blueberry Pancake Bites

Protein: 6g Fat: 13g Net Carbs: 7.5g Calories: 188 Fiber: 4g

Ingredients:

- ½ cup frozen blueberries
- 1/3 – ½ cup water
- ½ tsp. cinnamon
- 1 tsp. baking powder
- ¼ cup melted ghee
- ½ tsp. salt
- ½ cup coconut flour
- ½ tsp. vanilla extract
- 4 eggs

Instructions:

1. Ensure your oven is preheated to 325 degrees. With the butter and coconut oil spray, grease a muffin tin.
2. Mix the vanilla, sweetener, and eggs together until smooth.
3. Stir in the cinnamon, salt, baking powder, melted ghee, and coconut flour, blending till smooth.

4. To the batter, add 1/3 cup of the water and blend once more. The batter should be thick.
5. Among the muffin tin cups, divide the batter and then add a few blueberries to each muffin.
6. For 20 to 25 minutes, bake until set.
7. Allow to cool.

Can be kept in a slightly cold place in an airtight container for 8-10 days. Can be frozen for 60-80 days.

Lunch Recipes

Shredded Chicken for Meal Prep

Calories: 115 Sugar: 0g Carbs: 0g Total Fat: 4g Protein: 19g

Ingredients:

- ½ tsp. black peppercorns
- 2 bay leaves
- 2 halved cloves of garlic
- 32 ounces of chicken broth (preferably reduced-sodium)
- 4 ½ - 5 pounds skinned chicken thighs
- 4 parsley stems
- 4 thyme sprigs

Instructions:

1. Put the chicken in your slow cooker.
2. In a double-wrapped cheesecloth, place the peppercorns, garlic, bay leaves, parsley stems, and thyme sprigs. Tie off the cheesecloth and add the filled bouquet to the slow cooker.
3. Pour the broth into your slow cooker over the chicken and wrapped herbs.

4. Cover them and set to cook on low heat setting for 7 to 8 hours.
5. Discard the bouquet.
6. Place the chicken in a bowl and leave the cooking liquids in the cooker.
7. Once some of the chicken has cooled, take out the bones from the meat. Use two forks to shred the chicken, adding reserved cooking liquids while shredding to keep the meat moist.
8. Strain the remaining liquids and use for the future stock if desired.

Can be used in a large variety of meal prep recipes! To make ahead, place 2 cups of stock and chicken in separate containers.

Can be frozen for 3 months and refrigerated for 3 days.

Easy Sheet Pan Roasted Vegetables

*Calories: 97 Protein: 2g Carbs: 11g Total Fat: 6g
Sugar: 4g*

Ingredients:

- 1 tbsp. balsamic vinegar
- ¼ tsp. pepper
- 1 chopped red onion
- 1 tsp. coarse salt
- 2 chopped red bell peppers
- 2 tsp. Italian seasoning
- 3 tbsps. olive oil, extra virgin
- 3 cups cubed butternut squash
- 4 cups broccoli florets

Instructions:

1. Ensure your oven is preheated to 425 degrees.
2. Toss the cubed squash in a tablespoon of the oil and spread out onto a baking tray. Roast for 10 minutes.
3. Toss the pepper, salt, Italian seasoning, onion, bell peppers, and broccoli till coated well.

4. Add the roasted squash to the veggies. Toss well to incorporate. Spread the veggie mixture over two baking trays.
5. Roast for 17 to 20 minutes, making sure to stir around 1-2 times throughout the cooking process. Vegetables should be tender and browned in areas.
6. Drizzle with the vinegar before eating.

Can be refrigerated for up to 7 days.

Mango Coconut Chicken Bowls

Calories: 482 Sugar: 0g Carbs: 72g Total Fat: 8g Protein: 34g

Ingredients:

- ¼ cup sweetened shredded coconut
- 1 sliced avocado
- 2 cups cooked brown rice
- 4 chicken breasts (sliced lengthwise in half)

Mango marinade:

- 1 tsp. salt
- 2 tbsps. lime juice
- 1 tbsp. Sriracha
- 2 minced garlic cloves
- 1 tbsp. honey
- 2 tbsps. olive oil
- 1 mango

Corn salsa:

- ¼ cup cilantro
- 1 can drained black beans
- ½ diced red pepper
- ¾ tsp. salt
- 1 ½ cup corn

- 1 diced red onion
- 1 tbsp. lime juice

Instructions:

1. Ensure your oven is preheated to 425 degrees.
2. Cook the rice as per the package instructions.
3. In a blender, mix all of the mango marinade ingredients together till combined.
4. Marinate the chicken in half of the mango mixture for 10 minutes.
5. Mix together the corn salsa ingredients.
6. On your baking tray, place the chicken and bake for 15-20 minutes till golden in color.
7. Slice the chicken and place into bowls, along with additional mango sauce, corn salsa, topped with the shredded coconut and cilantro. Place the avocado on top.

Can be chilled in your fridge up to 5 days.

Chicken Tikka Masala Prep Bowls

Calories: 215 Sugar: 2g Carbs: 17g Total Fat: 9g Protein: 21g

Ingredients:

- 1 ½ pounds chicken breasts (cut into 1-inch pieces; boneless, skinless)
- 1 cup brown rice
- 1 diced onion
- ¼ cup cilantro
- 1 tbsp. lemon juice
- 1 tbsp. ginger, grated
- 1/3 cup heavy cream
- 2 tbsps. tomato paste
- 1 cup chicken stock, reduced-sodium
- 2 tbsps. unsalted butter
- 2 tsp. garam masala
- 28-ounce can diced tomatoes
- 2 tsp. chili powder
- 3 minced garlic cloves
- 2 tsp. turmeric

Instructions:

1. Cook the rice in 2 cups of water following the package directions.

2. In a skillet, melt the butter. With the pepper and salt, season the chicken. Then, with the onion, add the chicken to the skillet, cooking for 4 to 5 minutes till golden.
3. Stir in the turmeric, chili powder, garam masala, ginger, and tomato paste, cooking for 1 to 2 minutes as you combine.
4. Pour the chicken stock and tomatoes in. Bring the mixture to a boil.
5. Decrease heat. Then, for 10 minutes, let it simmer, stirring on occasion.
6. Mix in the lemon juice and cream, heating through 1 minute.
7. Spoon the rice and chicken into the meal prep bowls and garnish with the cilantro.

Refrigerated for up to 7 days or frozen for 1 month.

Spinach, Tomato, and Bacon Muffin Tin Quiche

Calories: 96 Carbs: 2g Sugar: 0g Protein: 13g Total Fat: 9g

Ingredients:

- ¼ cup tomatoes, diced
- ½ cup low-fat milk
- ½ tsp. pepper
- ½ cup chopped green onions
- ½ tsp. salt
- 1 ½ cup red-skinned potatoes, diced
- 2-ounces shredded cheese of choice
- 1 ½ cup chopped spinach
- 2 tbsps. extra virgin olive oil
- 3 strips of cooked/chopped bacon
- 8 eggs

Instructions:

1. Ensure your oven is preheated to 325 degrees. Liberally grease a muffin tin.
2. Set over medium heat, warm oil in a pan. To the pan, add some salt and potatoes, stirring for 5 minutes till the potatoes are just

cooked. Take it off the heat. Allow to sit and cool for 5 minutes.
3. Whisk the pepper, salt, milk, cheese, and eggs together.
4. Fold in the cooked potatoes, tomatoes, green onion, and spinach to the egg mixture.
5. Pour the egg and veggie mixture evenly in your muffin tin.
6. Bake for 25 minutes till firm to the touch.
7. For 5 minutes, allow to sit.

Can be refrigerated for 3 days and frozen up to a month.

To reheat, remove the plastic wrapper, put a dampened paper towel around it, and then heat in the microwave for 30 to 60 seconds. Enjoy!

Taco Scramble

Calories: 450 Carbs: 24g Sugar: 3g Total Fat: 19g Protein: 46g

Ingredients:

- ¼ cup chopped scallions
- ¼ cup water
- ¼ tsp. adobo seasoning salt
- ½ cup Mexican shredded cheese
- ½ minced onion
- 1 pound lean ground turkey
- 2 tbsps. homemade taco seasoning (Tastier and better for you than the store-bought!)
- 2 tbsps. minced bell pepper
- 4-ounce can tomato sauce
- 8 beaten eggs

Potatoes:

- ½ tsp. garlic powder
- 1 pound red potatoes, quartered
- ¾ tsp. salt
- 4 tsp. olive oil

Homemade taco seasoning:

- 1 tsp. chili powder

- ½ tsp. oregano
- 1 tsp. paprika
- 1 tsp. cumin
- 1 tsp. garlic powder
- 1 tsp. salt

Instructions:

1. Beat the eggs, add the seasoning salt, and fold in the cheese.
2. Ensure your oven is preheated to 425 degrees. Grease a casserole dish.
3. Add the oil, salt, garlic powder, and 1-2 pinches of the pepper to the potatoes. Bake the potatoes for 45 minutes till tender, making sure to stir every 15 minutes.
4. Brown the turkey. Then add the water, tomato sauce, bell pepper, and onion. Stir, simmering for 20 minutes
5. Spray a separate skillet liberally using the cooking spray and add the eggs and ¼ teaspoon of the salt. Scramble for 2 to 3 minutes.
6. When serving, put ¾ cup of the turkey and 2/3 cup of the eggs into a meal prep container or serving bowl. Divide the potatoes among each serving with 1 tablespoon of the cheese and scallions.

Chicken Sausage and Peppers

Calories: 249 Protein: 18g Carbs: 20g Total Fat: 11g Sugar: 11g

Ingredients:

- 1 sweet onion (cut into wedges)
- 2 cups grape tomatoes
- 1 tbsp. oregano
- 1 tbsp. vinegar, balsamic
- 12-ounce package of Italian-flavored cooked chicken sausage
- 1 tbsp. olive oil
- 4 sweet peppers, color of choice (chop into 1-inch pieces)

Instructions:

1. Ensure your oven is preheated to 425 degrees. Liberally grease a baking pan.
2. In the prepared pan, add the tomatoes, onion, and peppers. Drizzle with the vinegar and olive oil and toss. Roast for 30 minutes.
3. Move the roasted veggies to one side of the tray and put the sausage in an empty portion. Roast for another 10 to 15 minutes till the sausage is heated through.
4. Sprinkle with the oregano.

Can be refrigerated for 7 days and frozen for 15 days.

Southwestern Chicken Burrito Bowls

Calories: 301 Sugar: 3g Carbs: 10g Total Fat: 14g Protein: 21g

Ingredients:

- ¼ tsp. cayenne
- ¼ tsp. pepper
- 1 ½ cup canned black beans
- ½ tsp. cumin
- ¾ cup canned corn
- 1 cup grape tomatoes
- 1 cup cooked rice
- 1 tsp. paprika
- 2 cups kale
- 3 cups shredded chicken

Instructions:

1. Prepare the rice according to the package instructions. Mix the pepper, cayenne, cumin, and paprika in with the rice when there are around 5 minutes left to cook the rice.
2. Layer your meal prep containers with the shredded chicken, rice, beans, corn, kale, and tomatoes.

3. Top with the dressing and enjoy it right away or store in the fridge for later enjoyment.

Can be refrigerated for 7-10 days.

Skinny Joes With Tangy Slaw

Calories: 381 Protein: 29g Carbs: 23g Total Fat: 14g Sugar: 4g

Ingredients:

- 1 cup chopped tomatoes
- ½ cup rolled oats
- 1 cup water
- 1 red onion, chop
- 1 green or red bell pepper, chop
- 1 ½ tsp. salt
- 1 grated carrot
- 1 tbsp. Worcestershire sauce
- 1-pound ground beef, lean
- 2 tsp. garlic powder
- 1 tbsp. olive oil
- 4 tbsps. apple cider vinegar
- 4 tbsps. tomato paste

Tangy Slaw:

- ½ chopped red onion
- ½ head cabbage
- 1 tbsp. honey
- 1 tbsp. mustard, Dijon
- 2 grated carrots
- 2 tbsps. apple cider vinegar

Instructions:

1. Press SAUTÉ. Pour the oil into an instant pot and allow to heat for a bit. Add the beef and cook till browned.
2. Push the beef to the side in the pot and add the garlic powder, salt, carrots, peppers, and onions, sautéing for 5 minutes till softened. Then pour in the water, tomato paste, chopped tomatoes, vinegar, and Worcestershire sauce. Mix well to incorporate.
3. When the mixture heats to boiling, toss in the oats. DO NOT STIR.
4. Close the lid. Press HIGH PRESSURE. For 10 minutes, cook the mixture.
5. Perform the natural release. Let it sit for a few minutes covered to allow to thicken.

1. *To make the slaw*, combine the honey, vinegar, and mustard.
2. Add the onions, carrots, and cabbage, tossing with the honey mixture.

Sloppy joe meat can be frozen for up to 3 months and refrigerated for 10 days.

Tangy slaw can be refrigerated for up to 4 days.

Mason Jar Recipes

Asian Chicken Mason Jar Salad

Calories: 524 Sugar: 15g Carbs: 39g Total Fat: 33g Protein: 28g

Ingredients:

- 1 1/3 cup halved snap peas
- 1 cup grated carrots
- 1 cup whole cashews, unsalted
- 1 julienned red pepper
- 2 cups baby spinach, sliced
- 2 cups napa cabbage, sliced
- 1 1/3 cup sliced cucumber
- 2 cups shredded rotisserie chicken
- 2 tbsps. green onions, sliced

Sesame dressing:

- 1 minced garlic clove
- 2 tbsps. rice vinegar
- 1 tbsp. minced ginger
- 1 tbsp. honey
- 1 tsp. sriracha sauce
- 1 tsp. sesame seeds
- 2 tbsps. cilantro
- 1 tbsp. olive oil
- 2 ½ tbsps. sesame oil , toasted
- 3 tbsps. low-sodium soy sauce

- *4 64-ounce mason jars*

Instructions:

1. Whisk the sesame seeds, honey, cilantro, garlic, ginger, sriracha, olive oil, toasted sesame oil, vinegar, and soy sauce together.
2. Toss the spinach and napa cabbage together.
3. Assemble the jars by adding 3 tablespoons of the dressing, 1/3 cup of the snap peas, ¼ cup of the chicken, ¼ cup of the cashews, and a sprinkle of the green onion. Serve it now or place in the fridge. *Salads last 3 to 4 days in the fridge.*

Yogurt and Granola Parfait

Calories: 98 Sugar: 4g Carbs: 2g Total Fat: 4g Protein: 5g

Ingredients:

- 2 cups granola
- 2 cups Greek yogurt (any flavor)
- 4 cups berries

Instructions:

- Layer ½ cup of the granola, ½ cup of the yogurt, and 1 cup of the berries into the jar, continuously layering till you are out of ingredients.

Can be refrigerated for 3 to 4 days.

Zucchini Lasagna

*Calories: 114 Sugar: 4g Carbs: 3g Total Fat: 9g
Protein: 8g*

Ingredients:

- ¼ cup minced parsley
- ½ cup diced onion
- ½ pound lean ground turkey
- ½ tbsp. Italian seasoning
- ½ tbsp. minced garlic
- ½ tsp. oregano
- 1 cup part-skim mozzarella cheese
- 1 egg yolk
- 2 tsp. salt
- 1 tbsp. olive oil
- 2 zucchinis
- 6 tbsps. canned tomato sauce
- 4 tsp. parmesan cheese
- 6 tbsps. crushed tomatoes
- 8 ounces low-fat ricotta cheese

Instructions:

1. Ensure your oven is preheated to 350 degrees.
2. Slice the zucchinis 1/8-inch thick and sprinkle with 1 ½ teaspoon of the salt.

3. Bake for 15-25 minutes till the water is released from edges.
4. Lay the zucchini out on paper towels. Reduce the oven temperature to 325 degrees.
5. In a pan, warm the olive oil. Then pour turkey, garlic, and onion, cooking the meat till cooked through. Season with the seasonings. Set it aside.
6. Mix the crushed tomatoes and tomato sauce together. With the salt and pepper, season.
7. Mix the pepper, salt, egg, and ricotta together as well.
8. Layer half of the sauce between four jars. Then layer the turkey, zucchini noodles, and other ingredients. Parsley and mozzarella should go on top. Seal the jars well.

Can be refrigerated for 3 days.

Berry and Nuts Salad

Calories: 92 Sugar: 3g Carbs: 0.5g Total Fat: 7g Protein: 10g

Ingredients:

- ¼ cup chopped almonds
- ½ cup blackberries
- ½ cup blueberries
- ½ cup strawberries

Zesty Dressing:

- ¼ cup orange juice
- 1 tbsp. honey
- Juice and zest of a lemon
- 2 tbsps. olive oil

Instructions:

1. Whisk the dressing components together till blended.
2. In the mason jar, pour in 2-3 tablespoons of the dressing into the bottom. Then layer the berries, putting the almonds on the top.

Refrigerate for 3 days.

Asian Noodle Salad

Calories: 119 Sugar: 4g Carbs: 1g Total Fat: 5g Protein: 8g

Ingredients:

- ½ cup crunchy rice noodles
- 1 cup cooked/shelled edamame
- 4 green onions, sliced
- 2 carrots, peeled/shredded
- 4 ounces soba noodles

Spicy Peanut Dressing:

- ¼ cup olive oil, extra-virgin
- 4 tsp. vinegar, rice
- 2 tbsps. peanut butter
- 4 tsp. soy sauce
- 4 tsp. sambal

Instructions:

1. Whisk together all dressing components.
2. Pour the dressing into the bottom of the jar. Then layer the noodles, edamame, carrots, green onion, and noodles on top.

Refrigerate up to 4 days.

Mediterranean Salad

*Calories: 201 Sugar: 2g Carbs: 2g Total Fat: 4g
Protein: 13g*

Ingredients:

- 1 cup whole-grain couscous, cooked
- 1 tbsp. olive oil
- 2 ounces crumbles feta cheese
- 4-5 slices artichoke hearts, marinated in olive oil
- 6-10 cherry tomatoes
- Juice of ½ a lemon
- Sea salt
- Sprinkle of dried basil, oregano, and parsley

Instructions:

1. Mix all liquid ingredients together to create a type of the dressing.
2. Pour the dressing into the bottom of the jar. Then add other ingredients to the jar as you see fit.

Refrigerate for up to 3 days.

Feta and Shrimp Cobb Salad

Calories: 192 Sugar: 5g Carbs: 2g Total Fat: 8g Protein: 11g

Ingredients:

- 1 chopped hard-boiled egg
- 1-2 handfuls baby spinach and romaine lettuce
- 1 tbsp. chopped red onion
- 2 chopped slices bacon
- 2 tbsps. avocado
- 2 tbsps. chopped cucumber
- 2 tbsps. crumbled feta cheese
- 6-8 boiled shrimps
- 8 grape tomatoes
- Vinaigrette of choice

Instructions:

1. Pour the vinaigrette into the bottom of the jar.
2. Then layer the veggies, shrimp, bacon, and cheese on top.

Refrigerate for up to 4 days.

BLT Salad

Calories: 205 Sugar: 6g Carbs: 6g Total Fat: 18g Protein: 17g

Ingredients:

- 14 croutons
- 2 cups iceberg lettuce
- 2 cups romaine lettuce
- 2 chopped scallions
- 2 chopped tomatoes
- 4 crumbled slices bacon

Instructions:

1. Whisk all dressing components together.
2. Pour the dressing into the bottom of the jar.
3. Layer the veggies, then the croutons and bacon on top and seal.

Refrigerate for 3 days.

Rainbow Salad

Calories: 109 Sugar: 0g Carbs: 1g Total Fat: 9g Protein: 15g

Ingredients:

- ½ cup raw sunflower seeds
- 1 cup sliced carrots
- 1 cup cucumber, chop
- 1 bell pepper, yellow, chop
- 1 bell pepper, red, chop
- 2 cups chopped red cabbage
- 8 cups assorted salad greens

Balsamic Dressing:

- ¼ cup chopped parsley
- ½ cup white balsamic vinegar
- 2 minced cloves garlic
- Pepper and salt
- 2 tbsps. olive oil

Instructions:

1. Whisk all of the dressing components together.
2. Drain the chickpeas.

3. Pour the dressing into the bottom of the jar. Then layer the veggies and sunflower seeds on top. Seal well.

Can be refrigerated for up to 5 days.

Spinach, Tomato, Mozzarella Salad

Calories: 184 Sugar: 3g Carbs: 3g Total Fat: 12g Protein: 11g

Ingredients:

- 10 cups baby spinach
- 10 ounces fresh mozzarella
- 1-quart grape tomatoes
- 10 tbsps. balsamic vinegar dressing

Instructions:

- Pour the dressing in the bottom of the jar.
- Load the jar with the veggies and then the cheese. Seal well.

Can be refrigerated for up to 3 days.

Dinner Recipes

Chipotle Turkey and Sweet Potato Chili

Calories: 423 Carbs: 39g Total Fat: 18g Sugar: 6g Protein: 28g

Ingredients:

- ¼ - ½ tsp. ground chipotle powder
- 1 cup diced onion
- 1 tsp. oregano, dried
- 1 sweet potato
- 1 tbsp. oil, coconut
- 1 tsp. cumin
- 1-pound ground turkey
- 2 cups chicken broth
- 2 tsp. chili powder
- 28-ounces fire-roasted tomatoes
- 3 minced garlic cloves
- Pepper and salt

Instructions:

1. Warm up the coconut oil over intermediate-extreme warmth.
2. Once the oil begins to simmer, place the turkey in a pan. Cook for 5 minutes, breaking up as it cooks.

3. Toss in the garlic and onions, cooking for 8-10 minutes till the onions turn into translucent.
4. Turn the warmth up to high. Pour in the broth, sweet potato, and tomatoes, along with the seasonings. Bring the mixture up to a boiling point.
5. Turn down the heat to a medium setting and let simmer for 10-15 minutes uncovered. The longer you allow to simmer, the bigger the flavor.

Refrigerate for 7 days and freeze for up to 6 months.

Avocado Bacon Garlic Burger

Calories: 189 Sugar: 1g Carbs: 13g Total Fat: 22g Protein: 27g

Ingredients:

- ½ tsp. pepper
- 1 cup chopped basil
- 1 tsp. salt
- 1-pound grass-fed lean ground beef
- 2 eggs
- 3 minced cloves garlic

Toppings:

- 1 avocado
- 16 pieces of bacon, cooked
- 4 slices red onion

Instructions:

1. Mix all hamburger components till well incorporated.
2. Divide the meat into four patties.
3. In a pan, warm up the olive oil.
4. Then, place the patties, grilling for 4 minutes per side.

5. Make the burgers with the avocado as the bun and other desired toppings.

Chutney Cilantro Meatballs

Calories: 375 Sugar: 3g Carbs: 23g Total Fat: 29g Protein: 35g

Ingredients:

Sauce:

- ½ cup water
- 1 chopped yellow onion
- 2 tbsps. avocado oil
- 28-ounce can crushed tomatoes

Meatballs:

- ½ cup quick-cooking brown rice
- 1 tsp. salt
- 1 tsp. ras el hanout spice blend
- 1 pound ground turkey

Chutney:

- ¼ tsp. cayenne pepper
- 1 bunch cilantro
- 1 green onion
- ¼ tsp. pepper
- 1 tsp. sesame oil, toasted
- 1 tbsp. lemon juice

- ½ tsp. salt

Instructions:

1. To create the sauce, push SAUTÉ and warm up the oil. Sauté the onion for 10 minutes. Then add the water and tomatoes, mixing well as you heat to simmer.
2. To create the meatballs, mix the salt, ra el hanout, rice, and turkey together. Form the mixture into 12 meatballs.
3. Put the meatballs in an even layer in the simmering sauce, spooning a bit of the sauce over the meatballs.
4. Place the lid on, using the PRESSURE RELEASE to seal. Press CANCEL and select POULTRY for 15 minutes.
5. While the meatballs cook, prepare the chutney by combining all chutney ingredients together, grinding them into a paste with the mortar and pestle.
6. Perform the quick release on the meatballs. Serve in the sauce and top with the chutney.

Instant Pot Lamb Shanks

Calories: 338 Sugar: 6g Carbs: 19g Total Fat: 37g Protein: 42g

Ingredients:

- ¼ cup minced Italian parsley
- 1 cup bone broth
- 1 chopped onion
- 1 tbsp. balsamic vinegar
- 1 tsp. fish sauce, red boat
- 1 pound ripe Roma tomatoes
- 1 tbsp. tomato paste
- 2 chopped celery stalks
- 2 tbsps. ghee
- 3 pounds lamb shanks
- 2 chopped carrots
- 3 smashed/peeled garlic cloves
- Pepper and salt

Instructions:

1. Season with the shanks with the pepper and salt.
2. Press SAUTÉ on the instant pot, melt a tablespoon of the ghee. Place the shanks into the pot and sear on all sides for 8-10 minutes.

3. As the lamb browns, chop up the veggies. Take out the lamb from the pot.
4. Lower the heat and add the remaining ghee. To the pot, add the onion, celery, and carrots, seasoning with the pepper and salt.
5. Add the garlic cloves and tomato paste, stirring for at least 60 seconds.
6. Place the shanks back into the pot along with the tomatoes.
7. Pour the balsamic vinegar, fish sauce, and bone broth into the pot.
8. Lock the lid. Press MANUAL and set to cook for 50 minutes. Perform the natural release.
9. Remove the shanks to the plate and top with the sauce.

Cranberry Spice Pot Roast

Calories: 312 Carbs: 13g Total Fat: 29g Sugar: 16g Protein: 54g

Ingredients:

- ¼ cup honey
- ½ cup water
- ½ cup white wine
- 1 cup frozen whole cranberries
- 1 tsp. horseradish powder
- 2 cups bone broth
- 2 peeled garlic cloves
- 2 tbsps. olive oil
- 3 to 4 pounds of beef arm roast
- 3-inch cinnamon stick
- 6 whole cloves

Instructions:

1. Dry the meat with the paper towels. Season liberally with the pepper and salt.
2. Press SAUTÉ on the instant pot. Heat up the oil and place the roast in, browning for 8-10 minutes on all sides. Remove and put to the side.

3. Pour the wine into the instant pot. Using a wooden spoon, from the bottom, scrape the bits. Cook for 4-5 minutes to deglaze.
4. Add the cloves, garlic, cinnamon stick, horseradish powder, honey, water, and cranberries to pot. Cook for 4-5 minutes till the cranberries start to burst open.
5. Place the meat back into the pot. Pour in just enough bone broth to cover the meat.
6. Lock the lid. Press HIGH PRESSURE to cook for 75 minutes.
7. Perform the natural release of the pressure for 15 minutes and then quick release the rest.
8. Place the meat on the serving platter and top with the cranberry sauce.

Garlic Pork and Kale

Calories: 437 Sugar: 11g Carbs: 20g Total Fat: 31g Protein: 49g

Ingredients:

- 1 tsp. minced rosemary
- 1 tbsp. red wine vinegar
- 20-25 whole garlic cloves
- 2 sprigs of thyme
- 1 chopped yellow onion
- 2 tbsps. olive oil
- 2 ½ pound pork shoulder (boneless; cut into 1 ½-inch chunks)
- 2/3 cup red wine, dry
- 2/3 cup chicken broth

Instructions:

1. Season the pork liberally with the pepper and salt.
2. Press SAUTÉ on the instant pot and heat up the olive oil. Working in batches, sear the pork till browned. Remove with the slotted spoon. Discard the fat from the instant pot.

3. Add the thyme and onion to the instant pot, sautéing for 5 minutes. Then add the rosemary and garlic, cooking for 60 seconds.
4. Using a wooden spoon, pour wine in to deglaze the bits from the bottom of the pot.
5. Pour in the broth and add the pork back in. Combine.
6. Lock the lid. Press MANUAL to cook for around 40 minutes. Perform the quick release.
7. Stir in the kale. Press HIGH PRESSURE to cook for another 10 minutes. Perform another quick release.
8. Kale and pork should be nice and tender.

Can freeze up to 3 months.

Lemon Pepper Salmon

Calories: 174 Sugar: 1g Carbs: 29g Total Fat: 11g
Sodium: 118mg Protein: 36g

Ingredients:

- ¼ tsp. salt
- ½ thinly sliced lemon
- ½ tsp. pepper
- ¾ cup water
- 1 julienned carrot
- 1 julienned red bell pepper
- 1-pound salmon filet
- 1 julienned zucchini
- 3 tsp. ghee
- Few springs of basil, tarragon, dill, and parsley

Instructions:

1. Pour the herbs and water into the instant pot. Place a trivet into the pot and gently place the salmon onto it.
2. Drizzle the fish with the ghee, pepper, and salt. Cover with slices of the lemon.
3. Lock the lid. Press STEAM to cook for 3 minutes.

4. Julienne your veggies while the salmon cooks.
5. Perform the quick release. Press CANCEL. Remove the rack with the salmon.
6. Discard the herbs. To pot, add veggies. Press SAUTÉ and cook for 1-2 minutes.
7. Serve the salmon with the veggies, along with a teaspoon of the cooking fats if you so choose.

Beef and Broccoli

Calories: 259 Sugar: 2g Carbs: 12g Total Fat: 9g Protein: 28g

Ingredients:

- ¼ tsp. fresh ginger
- 1 tbsp. cooking oil
- 10 to 12-ounce flank steak or sirloin
- 2 minced garlic cloves
- 3 ½ cups broccoli florets
- water

Marinade:

- 1 tsp. cornstarch
- ¼ tsp. dark soy sauce
- ½ tsp. sesame oil
- 1 tsp. soy sauce, low-sodium
- 1/8 tsp. pepper

Sauce:

- ¼ tsp. dark soy sauce
- ½ tsp. dry sherry
- 1 tsp. sesame oil, toasted
- 1 ½ tbsp. oyster flavored sauce
- 1 ½ tsp. soy sauce, low-sodium

- 1/3 cup water, cold
- 2 tsp. cornstarch
- 2 tsp. sugar

Instructions:

1. Mix all marinade ingredients together. Add the beef slices and let them sit for at least 10 minutes.
2. Blanch the broccoli.
3. Combine all sauce ingredients together.
4. Warm the oil in either a pan or wok. Add the beef in a single layer to sear. Pour the garlic and continue cooking the meat till cooked through. Pour the sauce in, constantly stirring till it becomes thickened. Add more water to thin it out if needed. Add the broccoli and stir everything well to coat. Season with the pepper and salt if desired.
5. Sprinkle the sesame seeds and chopped onions if desired.
6. Divide among containers.

Shrimp With Zucchini Noodles

Calories: 119 Sugar: 1g Carbs: 4g Total Fat: 8g Protein: 14g

Ingredients:

- ½ pound shrimp
- 1 tbsp. olive oil
- 4 zucchinis, spiralized

Sauce:

- ¼ cup + 2 tbsps. Thai sweet chili sauce
- ¼ cup + 2 tbsps. light mayo
- ¼ cup + 2 tbsps. plain Greek yogurt
- 1 ½ tsp. sriracha sauce
- 1 ½ tbsp. honey
- 2 tsp. lime juice

Instructions:

1. Cook the shrimp till opaque.
2. Warm up the oil in a pan and add the zucchini till tenderized. Drain and let it rest for 10 minutes.
3. Mix all sauce components together until smooth.

4. Split up the sauce into the containers. Add the zucchini noodles and gently stir to coat well. Add in the shrimp among containers.

Shrimp Taco

*Calories: 215 Sugar: 1g Carbs: 3g Total Fat: 15g
Protein: 12g*

Ingredients:

Spicy Shrimp:

- ¼ tsp. onion powder
- ¼ tsp. salt
- ½ tsp. cumin
- ½ tsp. chili powder
- 1 tbsp. olive oil
- 1 clove garlic, minced
- 20 shrimps

For bowl assembly:

- ½ cup cheddar cheese
- 1 cup black beans
- 1 cup tomatoes
- 1 cup corn
- 1 lime
- 2 tbsps. cilantro

Instructions:

1. Mix all of the shrimp spices together. Add the shrimp, tossing gently to coat. Cover and chill for 10-15 minutes or up to 24 hours.
2. In a skillet, warm the oil and add the shrimp. Cook till cooked thoroughly.
3. To assemble the bowls amongst containers, top with five shrimps, a scoop of tomatoes, beans, corn, and a sprinkle of the cheese and cilantro and a lime wedge.

Refrigerate for up to 14 days.

Lemon Roasted Salmon With Sweet Potatoes and Broccolini

Calories: 223 Sugar: 3g Carbs: 5g Total Fat: 19g Protein: 19g

Ingredients:

- 1/8 tsp. red pepper flakes and thyme
- ¼ tsp. garlic powder
- Pepper and salt
- 2 tbsps. lemon juice
- 1 tbsp. butter
- 12 ounces of wild-caught salmon filets
- 4 cups broccoli florets
- 1-3 tbsps. olive oil
- ½ tsp. cumin
- 2 sweet potatoes, cubed

Instructions:

- Ensure the oven is preheated to 425 degrees. On a sheet pan, place the sweet potatoes on one side and the broccoli on the other. Drizzle both with the oil to the pepper, salt, and cumin and toss. Bake the potatoes for 15 minutes and put the broccoli to the side.

- Mix the pepper, salt, thyme, pepper flakes, garlic powder, lemon juice, and butter together. Heat for a few seconds in the microwave for the butter to melt.
- With the foil, line a tray, spray, and place the salmon on it. Drizzle the fish with the lemon sauce.
- Remove the potatoes, put the broccoli and salmon on the tray, and put back in the oven for another 12-15 minutes.
- Divide the veggies and fish among containers.

Dessert Recipes

Cinnamon Apples

Calories: 102 Carbs: 4g Total Fat: 3g Sodium: 24mg
Sugar: 32g Protein: 13g

Ingredients:

- ½ cup brown sugar
- 1 tbsp. cinnamon
- 2 tbsps. unsalted butter
- ½ cup sugar
- 1/8 tsp. nutmeg
- 3 tbsps. cornstarch
- 6 Granny Smith apples
- Pinch of salt

Instructions:

1. Peel and thinly slice the apples.
2. Pour all ingredients into your instant pot. Stir well to combine.
3. Press MANUAL to cook for 18 minutes. Perform the natural release.
4. Stir up the mixture well and serve!

Refrigerate for 7 days or freeze for 2 months.

Stuffed Peaches

Calories: 237 Sodium: 173mg Carbs: 8g Sugar: 36g Total Fat: 11g Protein: 15g

Ingredients:

- Pinch of sea salt
- ¼ tsp. almond extract
- ½ tsp. cinnamon
- 2 tbsps. butter
- ¼ cup maple syrup
- ¼ cup cassava flour
- 5 peaches
- ½ cup slivered almonds

Instructions:

1. Cut off about ¼ inch from the top of the peaches. Remove the pits and hollow them all out.
2. Mix together the remaining components till crumbly. Pour the crumble mixture into the peaches.
3. Place a steamer basket into the instant pot. Add 2 cups of the water and place the peaches into the basket.
4. Lock the lid, press MANUAL to cook for 3 minutes. Perform the quick release.

5. Remove the peaches and allow to cool for 10 minutes.

Can be refrigerated for 4 days.

Blackberry Curd

*Calories: 91 Sugar: 28g Carbs: 2g Total Fat: 0g
Sodium: 11mg Protein: 1g*

Ingredients:

- 2 tbsps. lemon juice
- 1 cup sugar
- 12 ounces fresh blackberries
- 2 egg yolks
- 2 tbsps. butter

Instructions:

1. Pour the lemon juice, sugar, and blackberries into an instant pot. Lock the lid. Press HIGH PRESSURE to cook for a minute.
2. For 5 minutes, perform the natural pressure release. Then quick release any remaining pressure.
3. Puree the blackberries and remove the seeds as best as you can.
4. Whisk the egg yolks and then add to the hot blackberry puree. Pour it back into the instant pot.
5. Press SAUTÉ and bring to a boil. Stir frequently. Turn off the instant pot and mix in the butter.

6. Pour into the storage container and allow to cool. Chill in the fridge until ready to eat!

Refrigerate for 7 days and freeze for up to 3 months.

Cinnamon Pecan Chia Bars

Calories: 175 Sugar: 9g Carbs: 15g Total Fat: 11g Sodium: 143mg Protein: 12g

Ingredients:

- ¼ cup almond butter
- ½ cup pecan pieces
- ¾ tsp. cinnamon
- 2 tbsps. chia seeds
- 12 Medjool dates, pitted

Instructions:

1. With the parchment paper, line a loaf pan. Allow the excess paper to hang over sides for easier removal later on.
2. In a blender, pour in all recipe components. Process till evenly distributed. The mixture should hold its shape.
3. In a loaf pan, pour mixture in. Firmly press into a block that is ½-inch thick. It will more than likely not take up the whole pan.
4. Chill for 45 minutes till the mixture has set. Slice into the bars.

Chocolate Coconut Bites

Calories: 71 Sugar: 1g Carbs: 21g Total Fat: 16g Sodium: 196mg Protein: 7g

Ingredients:

- ½ cup pecans
- 1 tbsp. cocoa powder
- ½ cup shredded coconut flakes, unsweetened
- 1 tbsp. milk, almond
- 1 tbsp. chia seeds
- 1 tbsp. collagen peptides
- 1 tbsp. liquid coconut oil
- 2 tbsps. hemp seeds
- 8 dates, pitted
- Extra coconut flakes (optional)

Instructions:

1. Blend all recipe components within a food processor till well incorporated.
2. Roll the mixture into 1-inch balls. Roll in additional coconut flakes if you so choose.

Freeze for up to 60 days.

Oatmeal Energy Bites

*Calories: 71 Sugar: 1g Carbs: 21g Total Fat: 16g
Sodium: 196mg Protein: 7g*

Ingredients:

- ½ cup almond butter
- ¼ cup ground flax seed
- 1 cup oats, rolled
- 1/3 cup honey, raw
- ½ cup chocolate chips

Instructions:

1. Mix all recipe components together.
2. Roll out teaspoon-sized balls onto a tray lined with the parchment paper.
3. Freeze the balls for 1 hour.

Freeze for up to 1 month.

Fat Bomb Recipes

Walnut Orange Chocolate Bombs

Calories: 87 Sugar: 1g Carbs: 2g Total Fat: 9g Protein: 2g

Ingredients:

- ¼ cup extra virgin coconut oil
- ½-1 tbsp. orange peel or orange extract
- 1 ¾ cup chopped walnuts
- 1 tsp. cinnamon
- 10-15 drops stevia
- 125 g 85% cocoa dark chocolate

Instructions:

1. Melt the chocolate with your choice of method.
2. Add the cinnamon and coconut oil. Sweeten the mixture with the stevia.
3. Pour in the fresh orange peel and chop the walnuts.
4. In a muffin tin or in the candy cups, spoon in the mixture.
5. Place in the fridge for 1-3 hours until the mixture is solid.

Mini Lemon Tart Bombs

Calories: 101 Protein: 3g Carbs: 1g Total Fat: 11g

Ingredients:

Crust:

- ¾ cup grated dried coconut
- 1 ½ tsp. vanilla extract
- 1 cup almond, cashew or other nut flour
- 2 tbsps. sugar substitute
- 3 tbsps. lemon juice
- 4 ½ tbsps. melted ghee
- Pinch of salt

Filling:

- ¼ tsp. salt
- 1/3 cup lemon juice
- ½ cup softened butter or ghee
- 1 tbsp. sugar substitute
- 1/3 cup full-fat almond or coconut milk
- zest of 2 lemons
- 1 tsp. sugar-free vanilla extract
- 2 tsp. lemon extract

Instructions:

1. *For the crust:* Combine entirely crust ingredients in a medium-sized bowl together. Then roll into a log shape with the help of the waxed paper.
2. Proceed to cut into 20-24 slices.
3. Roll each slice into a ball and press gently into the tart pans.
4. Chill until you are ready to fill the crusts.

5. *For the filling:* In a food processor, pour in the butter and beat till fluffy in the texture.
6. Add the salt, zest, extracts, sweetener, lemon juice, and milk, blending until smooth.
7. Taste the mixture periodically and add more lemon juice or sweetener until it meets your taste bud needs.
8. Then pour the filling into your frozen crusts.
9. Top with a sprinkle of the lemon zest.
10. Chill until the tarts are set. Should make about 24 tarts.

Cinnamon Roll Bomb Bars

Calories: 102 Carbs: 2g Total Fat: 15g Protein: 2g

Ingredients:

- ½ cup creamed coconut

- 1/8 tsp. cinnamon

First icing:

- 1 tbsp. butter, almond
- 1 tbsp. coconut oil, extra-virgin

Second icing:

- ½ tsp. cinnamon
- 1 tbsp. coconut oil (extra virgin) or almond butter

Instructions:

1. With the liners, line a mini loaf pan or baking dish.
2. Using your clean hands, combine the cinnamon and coconut cream. Then pat into a dish.
3. In a separate bowl, mix almond butter and coconut oil together. Then spread the mixture over the creamed coconut.
4. Place in the freezer for 5-10 minutes.
5. In yet another bowl, whisk together ingredients of second icing until combined. Drizzle the icing over bars and let it freeze again for 10-20 minutes.
6. Cut into bars and enjoy!

Can be frozen for up to 3 months.

Macadamia Chocolate Fudge Bombs

Calories: 267 Protein: 3g Carbs: 3g Total Fat: 19g

Ingredients:

- ¼ cup heavy cream or coconut oil
- 2 tbsps. sweetener of choice
- 2 ounces cocoa butter
- 2 tbsps. unsweetened cocoa powder
- 4 ounces chopped macadamias

Instructions:

1. In a saucepan, melt the cocoa butter over a simmering pot of water and then add the cocoa powder. Combine.
2. Pour in the sweetener and macadamia nuts and stir well.
3. Then add the cream, mixing well and bringing the mixture back to room temperature.
4. Pour the mixture into the molds or candy cups. Allow time for the bombs to cool and chill to harden.

Peanut Butter Chocolate Bombs

Calories: 211 Protein: 3.5g Carbs: 2g Total Fat: 15g

Ingredients:

- ¼ cup chopped walnuts
- ½ cup butter or coconut oil
- ½ cup natural peanut butter, plain or chunky
- ½ tsp. vanilla extract
- 1 cup sweetener of choice
- 1/3 cup powder, cocoa
- 2 ounces cream cheese, softened
- 1/3 cup vanilla whey powder
- Dash of salt

Instructions:

1. Line a 5 x 7 dish with the parchment paper, ensuring there is an overhang of paper of two sides to aid in the removal later on. Spread the melted butter over the paper as well.
2. In a saucepan on low heat setting, melt the butter and peanut butter together, combining well.

3. In another bowl, beat the cream cheese until it soft and proceed to beat in the peanut butter until smoothened mixture.
4. Add sugar substitute and vanilla.
5. Mix together the salt, protein powder and cocoa powder in a separate bowl, sifting dry ingredients into wet ones until smooth in texture. Stir in nuts.
6. Spread the fudge mixture into the prepared pan, placing in the freezer to harden.
7. Remove and cut into squares. Store in the chilled area before serving.

Savory Mediterranean Fat Bombs

Calories: 164 Protein: 4g Carbs: 2g Total Fat: 17g

Ingredients:

- ¼ cup butter or ghee
- ¼ tsp. salt
- ½ cup full-fat cream cheese
- 2 crushed garlic cloves,
- 2-3 tbsps. freshly chopped herbs
- 4 pieces of drained sun-dried tomatoes
- 4 pitted olives
- 5 tbsps. grated parmesan cheese

Instructions:

1. In a bowl, cut butter into tiny pieces. Then add cream cheese.
2. Let it sit in room temperature for 20-30 minutes until soft.
3. Mash together with the fork until mixed. Add the tomatoes and olives.
4. Add the garlic and herbs, and season to taste with the salt and pepper.
5. Mix well ingredients together.
6. Put in the fridge for 20-30 minutes until solidified.
7. Take out the mixture and form five small balls. Then proceed to the roll balls into the grated parmesan cheese.
8. Eat right away or store in the fridge.

Bacon Guac Bombs

Calories: 156 Protein: 5g Carbs: 1g Total Fat: 15g

Ingredients:

- 4 slices of bacon
- ¼ tsp. salt
- 1 tbsp. lime fresh lime juice
- ½ small diced onion
- 1 chopped chili pepper
- 2 cloves crushed garlic
- ¼ cup butter or ghee
- ½ large avocado
- 1-2 tbsps. freshly chopped cilantro
- 1/8 tsp. cayenne pepper

Instructions:

1. Ensure the oven is preheated to 375 degrees.
2. Using the parchment paper, line a baking tray and proceed to lay out the bacon slices, ensuring none overlap.
3. Cook the bacon for 10-15 minutes or until golden brown. Remove and let it cool.
4. In a bowl, mash together the remaining ingredients together until combined. Then add diced onion.

5. Add the bacon grease and combine. Cover the mixture with the foil and put into the fridge for 20-30 minutes.
6. Crumble the bacon to use as breading.
7. Roll the avocado mixture into about six balls and roll into bacon pieces.

Salmon Bombs

Calories: 147 Protein: 3g Carbs: 0.5g Total Fat: 16g

Ingredients:

- ½ cup cream cheese, full-fat
- 1 tbsp. lemon juice, fresh
- ½ package smoked salmon or smoked mackerel
- 1/3 cup butter
- 1-2 tbsps. chopped fresh or dried dill

Instructions:

1. In a food processor, pour in salmon, butter, and cream cheese, adding the lemon juice and dill while pulsing.
2. With the parchment paper, line a tray and place the salmon mixture in 2.5 tablespoon sizes on the tray.
3. Top with the dill and put in the fridge to chill for 1-2 hours until firm.

Jalapeno and Cheese Bombs

Calories: 142 Protein: 4g Carbs: 1g Total Fat: 15g

Ingredients:

- ¼ cup grated cheddar cheese
- ¼ cup unsalted butter
- 2 g halved, seeded, & chopped jalapeño peppers
- 3.5 ounces of full-fat cream cheese
- 4 slices of bacon

Instructions:

1. Ensure your oven is preheated to 325 degrees.
2. With the parchment paper, line a baking sheet, ensuring there is extra hanging over the edge to aid in removing later.
3. Mash together the cream cheese and butter in a bowl and then put in the food processor, mix until smooth in texture.
4. Lay out the bacon slices on the parchment paper, leaving a space between them. Cook for 25-30 minutes until the slices are crispy. Remove and set aside to allow to cool.

5. Add together the cheese and jalapeños to the cream cheese and butter mixture. Chill for half an hour to 1 hour until set.
6. Split up the mixture into six fat bombs and place them on the parchment paper. If serving right away, roll in the crumbled bacon. If later, chill the mixture before coating in the bacon.

Pizza Bombs

Calories: 112 Protein: 5g Carbs: 2g Total Fat: 10.5g

Ingredients:

- 14 slices of pepperoni
- 2 tbsps. freshly chopped basil
- 2 tbsps. sun-dried tomato pesto
- 4 ounces of cream cheese
- 8 pitted black olives

Instructions:

1. Chop up the olives and pepperoni.
2. In a bowl, mix all together the cream cheese, tomato pesto, and basil and add the pepperoni and olives, mixing well to combine.
3. Form the mixture into balls and then top with the pepperoni, basil, and olive.

Rice Alternatives

One of the toughest challenges when doing keto is finding substitutes for plain old white rice. Here's 10 easy ones.

Cauliflower Rice
Just mince up cauliflower to a rice-like consistency in a food processor and you're good to go. One serving even contains a day's worth of Vitamin C

Broccoli Rice
Same as above - also looks great for photos!

Green Bean Fries
Sauteed green beans with some garlic and olive oil go well with so many different meals.

Zucchini Noodles
A great way to add some more bulk to meals, ideal if you naturally need to eat a higher volume of food to stay full. Use a spiralizer to make these.

Butternut Squash Noodles
Same as above

...and the one food which isn't keto friendly - but everyone thinks is...

Quinoa!

Whether it's red, black or white quinoa, all of these have more than 30g of net carbs per serving, and as such, will usually break your state of ketosis. Avoid quinoa if you're doing keto.

Emergency Keto Meals at Popular Fast Food Chains

As much as we like to plan, it's not possible to stay consistent 100% of the time. Life gets in the way. Fortunately, most fast food chains now have keto friendly meals. Here's a few options at the big chains.

Subway

Skip the bread (duh) and opt for a salad instead. The tuna salad with cheese, black olives, green peppers, lettuce, spinach and pickles has just 330 calories and 7G net carbs. Don't bother with dressings or sauces outside of olive oil, salt and pepper - and you're good to go

Chipotle

A salad bowl with meat, tomato based salsa (no corn), sour cream and cheese is both delicious and keto-approved.

McDonald's

Pro-tip, you can order the sandwiches without bread! Some restaurants might give you a strange look. Worst case scenario you order normally and toss out the bun. The McDouble, McChicken and Grilled Chicken Sandwich are all keto friendly. As are the sausage and egg mcmuffins

Burger King

Same applies here, a Whopper or Double Cheeseburger without bread or ketchup is keto friendly.

Taco Bell

This one is a little more complicated - order a side of lettuce, side of beef, side of chicken, and side or two of guacamole, then combine for a quick and cheap meal.

KFC

Protein heaven over at the colonel. Grilled chicken thighs are 17g protein with 0 carbs per piece. Breasts are 38g with no carbs. You can also get a side of green beans.

Carl's Jr.

One of the few places which actually has Lettuce-wrapped as an option. The thickburger is just 9G of carbs when you opt for this keto-friendly choice.

Jimmy John's

Any of their sandwiches can be made as Unwiches (order a slim one if you want a save a few bucks) which means no bread.

Five Guys

Same as Carl's Jr. Just order the lettuce wrap options and you're good to go.

In-n-Out

Order your burger "protein style" - a hamburger, cheeseburger or double double comes it at 11G of net carbs with this method.

Chapter 5: Methods to Properly Store Food

Congratulations! So far you know the ins and outs of the ketogenic diet, meal prep mistakes to avoid, and a nice array of keto meal prep recipes to get you started! Now, it's time to discover the proper way to store your deliciously prepped meals so that you can enjoy them as if they were fresh off the press!

Pantry Tips

There are many other items besides fruits, veggies, and canned goods that can reside happily in a pantry. These tips pertain to the foods in storage that don't need to be frozen or refrigerated:

- To lengthen the time of prepper foods, store them in the plastic or glass meal prep containers

- Most canned foods that are low in acid, such as vegetables, crab meat, and tuna can last up to 2 to 5 years. Ensure you check the date.

- Canned foods that are high in acid, like the tomato-based items, pineapple, and grapefruit have a shelf life of 12 to 18 months.

- Conditions of storage areas should be cool, dark, and dry with temperatures that range from 50 to 70 degrees. Warm climate makes the food deteriorate faster, so keep the items away from the hot pipes, dishwasher, and oven.

Fridge Tips

- Stay alert for spoiled food. If anything looks or smells off, it should be thrown out. Yes, mold can happen in the fridge too.

- Keep the prepped meals covered and in the plastic or glass containers, wrapped in the foil or plastic wrap.

- Pay attention to the expiration dates.

- Be vigilant of the 2-hour rule of refrigeration, meaning not leaving items that require to be chilled out for more than 2 hours, such as dairy, seafood, eggs, meat, chicken, etc.

- Set the temperature in your fridge to 40 degrees or lower.

Freezer Tips

I want to nicely remind you that freezing meals does not kill bacteria, but it can stop it from growing. Most frozen foods can last for a long time, but the color, flavor, and tenderness of the frozen items can be affected the longer they are frozen.

- Thaw food in your fridge before prepping

- Don't fear the freezer burn; it's a quality of food issue, not a food safety problem

- Label all packages you freeze with the date, what food is in it, and any other identifying information that will help your meal prep efforts, such as what it weighs or how many servings are in the container

- Ensure that you properly wrap the food you wish to freeze, utilize the airtight storage containers, and use the bags, plastic wrap, and foil that is freezer-grade

- Set the temperature of your freezer to 0 degrees or below

Freezer vs. Fridge

Not all edibles are freezer friendly:

- Fruits high in water content
- Lettuce
- Uncooked batters
- Eggs
- Cooked pasta
- Soft cheeses
- Cultured dairy

Freeze your meals if you don't plan to consume them in 3 to 4 days after you prepare them. Remember that the prepping frozen meals take a bit more preparation time than refrigerated meals.

- Thaw out meals for a few hours or overnight before heating and consuming

- Frozen meals last substantially longer than refrigerated meals, some being able to be frozen up to 1 year

Refrigerated meals are capable of being tasty, fresh, and convenient for a few days. After prepping, you just have to nuke the meals in the microwave. After several days of living in the fridge, however, meals can lose their freshness, taste, and moisture. This is because dry air circulating takes the moisture out of the food.

Refrigerate the meals you plan to eat in 3 to 4 days.

Chapter 6: Meal Prep Kitchen Essentials

Setting the time aside each week to prep meals for the entire week is a great way to eliminate the cravings for unhealthy eats and keep you on the right track to achieving your health and fitness goals.

Many people avoid the task of meal planning and prepping simply because they think of it as another chore; this is because they are using the wrong kitchen tools to get this big job done. This chapter will share the essential tools you need to simplify the process of meal prepping and make it more manageable.

High-quality knives

One of the most crucial tools to meal prep is having a decent set of knives that allow you to slice, dice, chop, and chiffonade like a master chef! If you have dull knives in your kitchen drawers, you are *asking* for prepping disaster. Sharp knives will save you time and make meal prep a lot easier on your hands. I recommend stainless steel knives for longevity!

Measuring spoons and cups

If you are meal prepping around macro measurements, it's very crucial to ensure you are measuring correctly. Measuring cups can help you measure dry ingredients like nuts and seeds while measuring spoons will help measure spices.

Food scale

Even though the majority of people can easily get away with measuring with cups and spoons, there are some people that need to ensure accuracy with a food scale. These are also helpful to measure proteins.

Good kitchen utensils

Having good quality kitchen utensils is obviously essential for breezing through meal prep! When you have well-rounded utensils, you can better prepare a variety of meals with ease.

Cutting boards

Almost all meal prep recipes involve dicing, cutting, or chopping, so you need one of these at arm's length always.

Mixing bowls

Good mixing bowls are used to mix batters, marinate proteins, and much more.

Colander

Good for draining veggies and aiming for clean-tasting produce. You want crispy, rainbow-like vegetables, right?

Grater

Meal preppers love graters! It allows them to add lots of flavors to any recipe with a few simple swipes. Zest a lemon, shave some chocolate, grate a bit of nutmeg, etc.

Baking dishes

- Round cake pans
- 13 x 9 baking sheet
- 8 x 8 and 9 x 5 loaf pans
- Muffin pans
- Etc.

Non-stick skillet

Skillets are highly versatile, and you can cook just about anything in them with a little bit of fat.

Cast iron skillet

An amazing gadget for the keto diet, this skillet is capable of adding flavor and iron to your meals.

Sauté pans

Saucepan with lid

Sheet pans

Roasting pan

Cook an amazing evening meal that makes a ton of leftovers! You can even make extremely large batches of items such as granola.

Cooling rack

Spiralizer

Obviously regular pasta is not keto friendly, but a better, healthier alternative can be created with the help of spiralizing vegetables like zucchini. Yum!

Food Processor

Don't want to chop your veggies? Stick them in a food processor! Great for making pesto, hummus, dips, shredding chicken, etc.

Crockpot

Crock pots are a meal prepper's *dream* appliance; if you want to further your meal prep skills, you can save even *more* time with these babies and can make a large variety of meals and desserts.

High-speed blender

No matter if you are making the nut butter, sauces, soups, or smoothies, a good blender is a must and can help you blend in seconds!

Meal prep containers

Quality meal prep containers are an essential staple to the meal planning world. You want ones that are durable and that you can use consistently for a long period of time. Opt for containers with lockable lids rather than the standard lids which can fall off because of condensation.